THE CANCER FIGHTING DIET

A Beginner's Cookbook For Health And Wellness

Table of contents

Introduction to Cancer and Nutrition

Cancer is a complex and devastating disease that affects millions of people worldwide. It is caused by the uncontrolled growth of abnormal cells in the body and can spread and invade other tissues and organs.Factors that contribute to cancer development and progression, such as genetics and environmental exposures. There are many, but diet is one of the most important and modifiable risk factors.

In recent decades, an increasing number of studies have been conducted to understand the role of nutrition in cancer prevention and treatment. Many studies show that certain dietary patterns and specific nutrients can influence cancer development and progression, while others can help improve outcomes for cancer patients. It shows that it is possible.

One of the most important ways diet influences cancer risk is through its effect on inflammation. Chronic inflammation is a hallmark of cancer and can help cancer cells grow and spread. A diet high in processed foods, saturated fats, and added sugars can increase inflammation in the body, while a diet high in fruits, vegetables, whole grains, and lean protein reduces inflammation and reduces cancer risk.

Another way diet influences cancer risk is through its effects on hormones. Some cancers, such as breast and prostate cancer, are hormone sensitive and can be driven by certain hormones in the body. Diets high in animal fats and dairy can increase levels of these hormones, while diets high in plant foods lower hormone levels and help reduce cancer risk. In addition to reducing cancer risk, diet plays an important role in cancer treatment and survival. For example, cancer patients undergoing chemotherapy and radiation therapy often experience side effects such as nausea, vomiting, and loss of appetite. Eating a high-protein, nutrient-dense diet can support your body during treatment and improve outcomes can benefit from a healthy diet. A diet rich in fruits, vegetables, whole grains and lean protein can help reduce the risk of cancer recurrence and improve quality of life. and multifaceted. Although there is no one-size-fits-all approach to preventing or treating cancer through diet, there are many evidence-based recommendations that can help reduce cancer risk and improve outcomes. Choosing a healthy diet and incorporating a variety of nutritious foods into your diet can help reduce your risk of cancer and improve your overall health and well-being. and cancer are closely intertwined, and the relationship between the two is constantly being studied and explored. While much remains to be learned about the exact mechanisms behind the link between diet and cancer, certain dietary patterns and nutrients can help reduce cancer risk and improve outcomes for cancer patients.

One of the best-established associations between diet and cancer is the association between red and processed meat consumption and an increased risk of colon cancer. Studies consistently show that people who eat a lot of red and processed meat have a higher risk of colorectal cancer than those who eat less meat. The World Health Organization classifies processed meat as a carcinogen. This means that it can cause cancer.

Other diets that have been associated with an increased risk of cancer include diets high in saturated fat, added sugars, refined carbohydrates and low in fruits, vegetables, whole grains and fiber.

In contrast, diets high in plant foods, such as the Mediterranean diet and the Diet to Stop Hypertension (DASH) diet, are associated with reduced cancer risk and improved overall health.

Dietary habits can have a significant impact on cancer risk, but individual nutrients and phytochemicals in food also play an important role. For example, cruciferous vegetables such as broccoli, kale, and cauliflower contain a compound called sulforaphane, which has been shown to have anti-cancer properties. Similarly, antioxidant-rich fruits and vegetables (such as berries and leafy greens) may help reduce cancer risk by protecting cells from free radical damage.

A healthy diet not only reduces your risk of cancer, but it can also support your immune system, which is important in fighting cancer. A diet rich in nutrients and antioxidants can help support the immune system and improve outcomes for cancer patients. It is an important factor to consider in cancer prevention and treatment. By making healthy dietary choices and incorporating a variety of nutritious foods into your diet, you can reduce your risk of cancer and improve your overall health and well-being.

Chapter 1: Foods for a Cancer-Fighting Diet

Cancer is a disease that affects millions of people worldwide. Although there are many treatments for cancer, including chemotherapy, radiation therapy, and surgery, it is also important to eat a healthy, balanced diet. A cancer-fighting diet can help strengthen your immune system, reduce inflammation, and lower your risk of developing or recurring cancer.This chapter discusses foods that are beneficial to your cancer-fighting diet.

Fruits and Vegetables:

Fruits and vegetables are an essential part of a cancer-fighting diet. They are rich in vitamins, minerals and antioxidants that protect the body from cancer. Some of the best fruits and vegetables to include in your diet are:

Vegetables: Spinach, kale, collard greens, and Swiss chard are all rich in vitamins and minerals that help strengthen your immune system and help prevent cancer.

Cruciferous vegetables: Broccoli, cauliflower, cabbage and Brussels sprouts are all rich in cancer-fighting nutrients such as sulforaphane and indole-3-carbinol.

Citrus: Oranges, grapefruit, lemons and limes are rich in vitamin C, an antioxidant that helps prevent cancer.

Tomatoes: Tomatoes are rich in lycopene, a powerful antioxidant that helps prevent cancer, especially prostate cancer.

Whole grains:

Whole grains are a good source of fiber and may help reduce the risk of colon cancer. It also contains vitamins and minerals that strengthen the immune system. Some of the best whole grains to add to your diet include:
Oats: Oats are rich in dietary fiber, vitamin E and zinc.

Quinoa: Quinoa is a complete protein and is also rich in fiber, iron and magnesium.

Whole grain bread: Whole grain bread, pasta and crackers are all rich in fiber, iron and B vitamins.

Healthy Fats:

Healthy fats are an important part of a cancer-fighting diet. They help reduce inflammation in the body and help prevent cancer. Some of the best sources of healthy fats are:

Seeds: Chia seeds, flax seeds and hemp seeds are excellent sources of healthy fats, fiber and protein.

Avocado: Avocados are rich in healthy fats, fiber, vitamins and minerals.
Olive Oil: Olive oil is a great source of healthy fats and antioxidants.

Protein:

Protein is important for maintaining a healthy immune system and is important in the fight against cancer. The best protein sources for a cancer-fighting diet include:

Fish: Oily fish such as salmon and tuna are rich in omega-3 fatty acids, which help reduce inflammation in the body.

Red Meat: Red meats such as chicken and turkey are good sources of protein and low in saturated fat. is also important to consider. A diet high in processed foods, saturated fats, and added sugars may increase the risk of cancer and other chronic diseases. A diet high in whole, unprocessed foods can help reduce cancer risk and improve overall health.
Here are some other cancer-fighting diet tips. Try to include different colors in your diet. B. Red, orange, yellow, green, blue, purple.

Limit red and processed meat: Eating too much red and processed meat can increase your risk of colon and other cancers. Limit your intake of these foods and instead choose leaner protein sources such as chicken, fish and beans. They are often high in added sugars, unhealthy fats, and other additives that can increase your risk of heart disease and other chronic diseases. Choose whole grains, fruits and vegetables, nuts and seeds, as many unprocessed foods as lean protein sources.

Drink lots of water: Staying hydrated is important for overall health, including cancer prevention. Drink at least 8 glasses of water a day. Drink more water if you are active or live in a hot climate.

Limit Alcohol Consumption: Excessive alcohol consumption can increase the risk of several types of cancer, including breast, colon, and liver cancer. If you drink alcohol, do so in moderation (women, no more than 1 drink a day for her, and men, no more than 2 drinks a day for her).

By following these tips and incorporating cancer-fighting foods into your diet, you can reduce your risk of cancer and improve your overall health and well-being. Always talk to your doctor or registered dietitian if you have questions about diet and how it can help prevent cancer.

A cancer-fighting diet should be high in fruits and vegetables, whole grains, healthy fats and protein. It is important to choose a variety of foods from each of these groups to ensure that you are getting enough of them. It may also help reduce the risk of cancer. However, certain foods and ingredients can increase the risk of cancer or worsen existing conditions. In this chapter, we examine foods to avoid in a cancer-fighting diet.

Processed meats
Processed meats such as bacon, ham, sausages and hot dogs are high in saturated fat and salt and may increase your risk of cancer. Studies have linked processed meat to colon, stomach, and pancreatic cancers. Additionally, processed meats often contain preservatives such as nitrates and nitrites, which can form carcinogenic compounds in the body.

Red meat

Red meats such as beef, pork and lamb are also high in saturated fat and may increase your risk of cancer. Studies have linked red meat to colon, pancreatic, and prostate cancer. To lower your risk of cancer, they recommend limiting red meat consumption to three servings per week. Carbohydrates can cause inflammation in the body, increase insulin resistance, and lead to the development of cancer. Additionally, sugar may promote the growth and spread of cancer cells. To reduce your risk of cancer, it is recommended that you limit your consumption of sugar and refined carbohydrates and choose whole grain options instead. , has been associated with an increased risk of several types of cancer, including breast, liver, and esophageal cancer. Additionally, alcohol can damage DNA, leading to mutations and the development of cancer. To lower the risk of cancer, it is recommended that women limit their alcohol intake to one drink per day and men to two drinks per day.

Fried and grilled foods

Fried and grilled foods such as French fries, roast chicken, and grilled meats may contain carcinogenic compounds such as acrylamides and heterocyclic amines (HCAs). In addition, high fat content in fried foods may increase the risk of cancer. To reduce the risk of cancer, they recommended limiting consumption of fried and grilled foods and choosing low-temperature cooking methods such as steaming and baking. A type of saturated fat that has been chemically modified to increase stability and extend shelf life. Trans fats are found in many processed foods, including snack foods, baked goods, and fried foods.Studies have linked trans fats to an increased risk of several types of cancer, including breast and colon cancer. ing. To reduce the risk of cancer, they recommended avoiding foods containing trans fats and choosing foods high in healthy fats, such as nuts, seeds and avocados. High intakes can increase the risk of some types of cancer, including stomach and esophageal cancer. Additionally, salt may promote the growth of cancer cells. To reduce the risk of cancer, they recommend limiting salt intake and choosing low-sodium options. It is controversial regarding its potential link to sex and cancer. Although research has not clearly shown a link between artificial sweeteners and cancer, it is recommended that you limit your intake of artificial sweeteners and choose natural sweeteners such as honey or maple syrup instead.

In summary, a cancer-fighting diet should include a variety of nutritious foods while avoiding foods that may increase cancer risk. The above foods are just a few examples of what to avoid, but there may be other foods and ingredients specifically tailored to your individual needs and medical history.

Remember that you have the potential to give. Instead of trying to eliminate these foods from your diet entirely, focus on healthier choices and moderation. For example, instead of cutting out red meat entirely, choose lean cuts and limit consumption to a few times a week. It is also important to note . Other lifestyle factors, such as regular exercise, maintaining a healthy weight, and avoiding tobacco use, may also help reduce the risk of cancer. If you are, or are concerned about your cancer risk, talk to your doctor or licensed dietitian about how to get the most out of your diet and lifestyle to reduce your risk.

Chapter 2: Meal Planning for a Cancer-Fighting Diet

Meal planning is an important aspect of a cancer-fighting diet. By planning your meals in advance, you can make sure you are on track, have a balanced and nutritious diet, and make meal times more manageable. Learn the basic principles of a meal plan to combat .

Eat colorful fruits and vegetables

Fruits and vegetables are the foundation of a cancer-fighting diet. Fill them with vitamins, minerals, fiber and antioxidants that help protect the body from cancer. It's important to include a variety of colored fruits and vegetables in your diet to ensure you're getting a variety of nutrients. Aim to eat at least five servings of fruits and vegetables a day.

Choose Whole Grains

Whole grains are another essential part of a cancer-fighting diet. They are rich in fiber, vitamins, minerals, and phytochemicals that help reduce cancer risk. Examples of whole grains include brown rice, quinoa, whole grain bread, and oatmeal. Choose whole grains over refined grains such as white bread, pasta, and rice.

Include Lean Protein Sources

Protein is essential for building and repairing tissues in the body. However, not all protein sources are created equal.Choose lean protein sources such as chicken, turkey, fish, beans, lentils, and tofu. Red meat, processed meat, and high-fat dairy products should be limited or avoided altogether.

Incorporate Healthy Fats

Healthy fats, found in avocados, nuts, seeds and fatty fish, can help reduce inflammation and promote overall health. However, it is important to eat in moderation as it is high in calories.
Reduce processed foods and sugar. Try to limit your intake of processed foods such as fast foods, packaged snacks, and sugary drinks. Instead, focus on whole foods that are minimally processed.

Hydrate with Water

Drinking enough water is very important for your overall health, especially if you are fighting cancer. Water flushes toxins from your body and keeps your digestive system working properly. Aim to drink at least eight glasses of water a day. Start planning your meals for the week ahead. Find recipes that include cancer-fighting foods and create a shopping list of the ingredients you need. Consider preparing meals in bulk and freezing them later in the week. With healthy meals on hand, you can resist the temptation to order takeout or eat ready-made meals. Meal plans are helpful, but it's important to be flexible. Life happens and sometimes plans change. If you don't have time to prepare meals, make a backup plan. B. Healthy frozen meals or simple sandwiches. Don't blame yourself if you accidentally eat something you didn't plan to eat. Get back on the road with your next meal.

Breakfast Ideas

Breakfast is the most important meal of his day and a great time to incorporate cancer-fighting foods into his diet. A nutritious breakfast should contain protein, healthy fats and whole grains. Here are some ideas for cancer-fighting breakfasts:

Oatmeal with fresh berries, nuts, and seeds

Greek yogurt with sliced fruit and granola

Scrambled eggs with whole-grain toast and avocado

Smoothie made with spinach, banana, berries, and almond milk

Lunch Ideas

Lunchtime can be challenging when you're on-the-go, but it's still possible to make healthy choices. To ensure that you're getting a balanced meal, include lean protein, whole grains, and plenty of vegetables. Here are some ideas for cancer-fighting lunches:

Quinoa bowl with roasted vegetables and grilled chicken

Salad with mixed greens, grilled salmon, avocado, and nuts

Whole-grain wrap with hummus, vegetables, and turkey or tofu

Lentil soup with a side of whole-grain bread

Dinner Ideas

Dinner is an excellent opportunity to prepare a delicious and healthy meal for yourself and your family. To ensure that you're getting a balanced meal, include lean protein, whole grains, and plenty of vegetables. Here are some ideas for cancer-fighting dinners:
Grilled chicken or fish with roasted vegetables and sweet potato

Stir-fry with tofu, brown rice, and vegetables

Baked salmon with quinoa and steamed broccoli

Turkey chili with a side of whole-grain bread and salad

Snack Ideas

Snacking can be a healthy addition to your diet, as long as you choose the right foods. Choose nutritious snacks that keep you feeling full and satisfied.

Apple wedges and almond butter

Carrots and hummus

Greek yogurt with berries and nuts

Popcorn with nutritional yeast and spices

Trying to stick to a cancer-fighting diet and when. But it's still possible to make healthy choices. Here are some dining tips:

Look for restaurants that offer healthy options like salads, grilled protein and vegetable garnishes.

Check the menu online before planning your meals in advance.

Ask for dressings or sauces on the side so you can control how much you eat.

Avoid fried foods and foods high in sugar and fat.

Share with friends and family to reduce portions.

In summary, a meal plan is essential to adopting a cancer-fighting diet. A balanced, nutritious diet that helps reduce the risk of cancer by eating a variety of colorful fruits and vegetables, whole grains, lean proteins, healthy fats, and limiting processed foods and sugar. can be made. Remember to plan, be flexible, and enjoy your journey to a healthier lifestyle.

Chapter 3: A Simple, Easy Breakfast to Fight Cancer

The adage that "breakfast is the most important meal of his day" applies to fighting cancer. A nutritious start to the day not only provides your body with the energy it needs, but it also helps keep your immune system strong.

Berry Nuts Overnight Oats

Overnight Oats are great for those who don't have time in the morning. Simply mix oatmeal, almond milk, chia seeds, and honey in a jar and refrigerate overnight.In the morning, top with fresh berries and a handful of nuts, such as walnuts or almonds.Nuts are a great source of healthy fats and protein. Despite being a poor source, berries contain antioxidants.

Avocado Toast with Smoked Salmon

Avocado toast has become a breakfast favorite, and with good reason. Avocados are rich in healthy fats, fiber and vitamins, and smoked salmon is a great source of protein and omega-3 fatty acids. To prep, toast a slice of whole wheat bread and sprinkle with avocado puree, smoked salmon and black pepper.

Greek Yogurt Parfait with Fruits and Nuts

Greek yogurt is an excellent source of protein, paired with fresh fruit and nuts for a hearty breakfast. Layer Greek yogurt, mixed berries, and chopped nuts in a parfait glass or bowl.Add a touch of honey or maple syrup for added sweetness.

Quinoa Bowl with Roasted Vegetables and Eggs

Quinoa is a versatile and nutritious grain that can be used in a variety of dishes, including breakfast bowls. Cook the quinoa according to package directions and serve with roasted vegetables such as sweet potatoes or brussels sprouts. Finish with a fried egg or two for extra protein. It's a quick and easy way to pack a lot of coffee, but it's even better with a smoothie bowl. Whisk spinach, frozen berries, almond milk and 1 tablespoon of protein powder until smooth. Pour into bowls and top with fresh berries, nuts and granola.

Veggie Omelette on Whole Wheat Toast

Eggs are a great source of protein and can be cooked in many ways. A vegetarian breakfast includes an omelet with spinach, mushrooms and diced tomatoes. Serve with a slice of whole wheat toast for extra fiber. Scrambled eggs are whipped with black beans and salsa and wrapped in whole wheat tortillas. Garnish with sliced avocado and sprinkle with cheese for extra flavor.

Incorporating these quick and easy breakfast ideas into your daily routine will help you get your day off to a good start. Choose whole foods that are nutritious and aim for a balanced diet that includes protein, healthy fats and fiber. Changing your breakfast routine can set you up for a healthier, cancer-fighting day.

Here are some other options that you can easily incorporate into your cancer-fighting diet.
Berry Almond Chia Pudding

Chia seeds are an excellent source of dietary fiber, healthy fats and antioxidants. For chia pudding, mix chia seeds with almond milk and refrigerate overnight. Garnish with fresh berries in the morning and sprinkle with crushed almonds for extra crunch.

Banana Peanut Butter Smoothie

Bananas are a good source of potassium, while peanut butter provides protein and healthy fats. Combine frozen bananas, peanut butter, almond milk and a little protein powder for a quick and filling breakfast smoothie.

Cottage Cheese with Fresh Fruit

Cottage cheese is a great source of protein and can be paired with a variety of fruits for a healthy breakfast. Try cottage cheese with sliced peaches, kiwi, or pineapple for a sweet and tangy breakfast option.
Oatmeal with Cinnamon and Apple

Oatmeal is high in fiber and can be easily customized with a variety of toppings. Try adding a sliced apple and a pinch of cinnamon to your oatmeal for a cancer-fighting breakfast. Apples are rich in antioxidants, while cinnamon has anti-inflammatory properties.

Boiled Egg Breakfast Salad

Salads aren't just for lunch and dinner. A breakfast salad is a great way to get a variety of nutrients in one meal. Try combining spinach, sliced strawberries, and hard-boiled eggs for a high-protein breakfast salad. Topped with a simple olive oil and balsamic vinegar vinaigrette.

Sweet Potato Hash with Eggs

Sweet potatoes are a great source of beta-carotene and can make a delicious breakfast hash. Cook diced sweet potatoes in a skillet with your favorite onions, garlic and spices. Serve with a fried egg or two for extra protein.

Chapter 4: Cancer-Fighting Lunch Nutrition

Lunch time can be a difficult time for many people, especially when trying to eat a healthy cancer-fighting meal. It's easy to find quick and convenient options, but these options often lack nutrients to fuel your body and fight cancer. In this chapter, we explore delicious and nutritious lunch ideas to help you stay on track with your cancer-fighting diet.

Grilled Chicken Salad

Grilled Chicken Salad is a delicious and hearty lunch that is easy to customize to your liking. Start with a bed of leafy greens like spinach, kale, and arugula, then add sliced cucumber, cherry tomatoes, and sliced carrots. Topped with grilled chicken breast and served with a homemade dressing made with olive oil, lemon juice and Dijon mustard.

Lentil Soup

Lentil Soup is perfect for those looking for a warm and comforting lunch. Lentils are a great source of protein and fiber, which can help keep you feeling full and satisfied.To make the soup, stir chopped onions, carrots and celery in olive oil until soft. . Add vegetable or chicken broth, lentils, or other vegetables of your choice. B. Chopped diced tomatoes or spinach. Cook until the lentils are cooked and season with salt and pepper.

Tuna Salad Wrap

Tuna Salad Wrap is a portable lunch that's easy to take on the go. First, mix canned tuna with Greek yogurt, Dijon mustard, diced celery, and red onion. Spread mixture on whole wheat wrap and add sliced avocado and leafy greens.Roll up and enjoy!

Quinoa and Black Bean Bowl

Quinoa and Black Bean Bowl is perfect for those looking for a plant-based lunch rich in protein and fiber. Start by cooking the quinoa according to package directions, then add black beans, diced tomatoes, diced avocado, and chopped coriander. Homemade dressing made with lime juice, olive oil, and cumin. Sprinkle on to add flavor.

Grilled Vegetable Sandwich

Grilled Vegetable Sandwich is a delicious addition to your veggie lunch. Grill sliced eggplant, zucchini, and peppers until tender and lightly browned. Spread hummus on whole grain bread and add grilled vegetables, leafy greens and chopped tomatoes. Season with salt and pepper.

A healthy, nutritious lunch is an important part of a cancer-fighting diet. Incorporating these delicious and nutritious lunchtime ideas into your daily routine can give your body the energy to fight cancer and maintain optimal health. Remember to choose whole foods rich in antioxidants, fiber and protein to keep you feeling satisfied.

When fighting cancer, it's important to focus on providing your body with foods rich in nutrients, vitamins and minerals. This is especially true at lunchtime when we often rely on convenience foods that can be high in calories, fat and sugar.

All of the above lunch ideas are nutritious and designed to fight cancer, with a focus on whole, unprocessed foods.Chicken breast is a lean, healthy protein. source, our grilled chicken salad is perfect for those looking for a high-protein lunch. Rich in fiber and nutrients, lentil soup is perfect for those looking for a warm and comforting lunch.

Avocado and Greek Yogurt Tuna Salad Wraps are a great way to incorporate healthy fats into your diet. Quinoa and black bean shells are a plant-based option rich in protein, fiber and antioxidants.Finally, grilled veggie sandwiches are a delicious way to eat veggies and are easy to customize with your favorite veggies.

When preparing lunch, try to focus on whole foods and avoid processed and packaged foods that are high in preservatives, additives and artificial ingredients. A diet rich in fruits, vegetables, whole grains, and lean protein can help provide your body with nutrients to fight cancer and maintain optimal health. In addition, remember to drink plenty of water throughout the day and avoid sugary drinks like sodas and fruit juices. Healthy snacks like nuts, seeds, and fruit also help keep you feeling full and satisfied.

By focusing on nutritious, cancer-fighting foods during your lunch break, you can support your body's natural defenses and maintain optimal health.

Chapter 5: A Satisfying Dinner to Fight Cancer

Dinner is the time when many of us sit down and enjoy a meal with our loved ones. It's time to unwind and nourish your body with healthy, nutritious food.

Grilled Salmon with Roasted Vegetables
Grilled salmon is a rich source of omega-3 fatty acids that have been shown to have anti-cancer properties. Pair with a variety of grilled vegetables for a hearty meal. To prepare this dish, first preheat your grill or grill pan. Brush the salmon with olive oil, lemon juice and a mixture of herbs and spices of your choice. Grill salmon on one side for 5 to 6 minutes, or until fully cooked. Meanwhile, toss vegetables of your choice (broccoli, green peppers, sweet potatoes, etc.) with olive oil, salt, and pepper. Roast vegetables in a 200°F oven for 25 to 30 minutes or until tender and golden brown. Serve salmon and vegetables together for a delicious and healthy dinner.

Lentil and Vegetable Stew

Lentils are a good source of vegetable protein and fiber, which may help reduce the risk of many types of cancer. This hearty lentil and vegetable stew is perfect for a filling dinner. To prepare this dish, first sauté onions, garlic, and your favorite vegetables (carrots, celery, peppers, etc.) in a large pot. Add canned diced tomatoes, lentils, vegetable stock, and your favorite herbs and spices. Simmer the stew for 20-30 minutes or until the lentils are tender and the flavors have melded. Serve the stew with a side salad or crusty whole wheat bread for a complete meal. It's also a great source of vitamins and minerals that help fight cancer. This zucchini noodle skillet is a delicious and easy-to-make dinner option. To prepare this dish, first sterilize the zucchini into long, thin noodles. Heat a large skillet over medium-high heat and add the olive oil. Saute the sliced bell peppers, mushrooms and garlic until soft. Add the zucchini noodles to the pan and cook 2-3 minutes or until medium hot. Dip it in your favorite stir-fried sauce (soy sauce, zizu sauce, sesame oil, etc.) and enjoy it piping hot.

Black Bean and Avocado Baked Sweet Potatoes
Sweet potatoes are an excellent source of beta-carotene, which has been shown to have anti-cancer properties. This easy baked sweet potato with black beans and avocado is a delicious and

filling dinner option. To prepare this dish, first he preheats the oven to 400°F. Prick the sweet potatoes with a fork in several places and arrange them on a baking sheet. Bake sweet potatoes for 45 to 50 minutes or until soft and caramelized. Meanwhile, heat a can of black beans in a small saucepan. Mash the avocado with lime juice, salt and pepper. Cut a sweet potato in half and top with black beans and mashed avocado. Serve hot.

Quinoa and Vegetable Salad

Quinoa is a nutritious grain rich in protein and fiber. This quinoa and vegetable salad is a delicious and healthy dinner option for hot summer nights.
To prepare this dish, first cook the quinoa according to package directions. While the quinoa is cooking, chop various vegetables such as cucumbers, cherry tomatoes, green peppers, and red onions. Once the quinoa is ready, place it in a large mixing bowl and add the chopped vegetables. Drizzle with olive oil and lemon juice, and season with salt and pepper. Toss everything together until well blended. Fresh herbs such as parsley and coriander can also be added for added flavor and nutrition.Serve the quinoa and vegetable salad chilled or at room temperature as a main course or side dish.

Grilled Chicken and Vegetable Skewers
Grilled chicken is a great source of protein and a favorite of many. Combined with a variety of colorful vegetables, it makes for a complete and satisfying cancer-fighting dinner. To prepare this dish, start by marinating the chicken breast in your favorite marinade for at least an hour. Cut vegetables of your choice into bite-size pieces (zucchini, red onions, cherry tomatoes, green peppers, etc.). Skewer chicken and vegetables alternately. Preheat a grill or griddle and cook skewers 8 to 10 minutes per side or until chicken is seared. Serve piping hot chicken and vegetable skewers with brown rice or salad.

Vegetable and Bean Chili
Hearty chili makes a hearty and filling dinner, especially during the colder months. They stuffed this vegetable and bean chili with anti-cancer ingredients such as tomatoes, beans, and various colorful vegetables. carrots, peppers, zucchini, etc.) in a large pot. Add canned diced tomatoes, vegetable broth, beans (such as black beans or kidney beans), and your favorite chili seasoning (chili powder, cumin, paprika, etc.). Simmer peppers for 30 to 40 minutes or until flavors are blended and vegetables are tender. Serve chili hot

with whole wheat bread or crackers. They've
packed these seven satisfying dinners with cancer-
fighting nutrients, flavors, and textures. Experiment
with different herbs, spices, and vegetables to
create your own delicious cancer-fighting dinner
recipes. please. Also, with portion sizes in mind,
remember to balance your meals with different
foods from different food groups for optimal
nutrition.

Chapter 6: Tasty Snacks and Appetizers to Fight Cancer

You can also protect your body by choosing the right snacks and appetizers. These small but important decisions can have a huge impact on your overall health and well-being.So let's dive into delicious and nutritious options!

Hummus with Vegetables

A great source of protein and healthy fats, hummus is incredibly versatile. Serve with sliced carrots, cucumbers, bell peppers, or any other vegetable of your choice. You can also use whole grain flatbreads or crackers for dipping.

Avocado Toast

Avocado Toast is a nutritious and trendy snack. Avocados are rich in healthy fats and antioxidants, and whole grain breads provide fiber and complex carbohydrates.Tossed with cherry tomatoes, diced onions, or flaxseeds for even more cancer-fighting benefits.

Greek Yogurt with Berries

Greek Yogurt is a great source of protein and pairs great with fresh berries like strawberries, blueberries and raspberries. They've packed the berries with antioxidants that help fight cancer-causing free radicals.

Quinoa Salad

Quinoa is a complete protein, rich in fiber and antioxidants. Enjoy with your favorite vegetables such as cherry tomatoes, cucumbers, and green peppers. Nuts and seeds such as walnuts and pumpkin seeds can also be added for crunch. Toss with olive oil, lemon juice and herb vinaigrette dressing.

Roasted Sweet Potato Fries

Sweet Potatoes are an excellent source of dietary fiber, beta-carotene, and vitamins A and C. Cut into fries and toss with a little olive oil, salt and pepper.

Bake in the oven until crisp and golden. Dip in some homemade aioli or guacamole for added flavor.

Edamame

Edamame is a soybean rich in protein, fiber and antioxidants. Steam until the pods are soft and sprinkle with a little salt. It can also be toasted in the oven for a crunchy texture. Serve them as a snack or appetizer and invite guests to take them out of the pod. Sliced whole wheat baguette with diced tomatoes, basil, garlic and a drizzle of olive oil.

Tuna Salad Salad Wrap

Tuna is an excellent source of lean protein and pairs well with fresh vegetables and herbs. Mix canned tuna with diced celery, onion, and parsley. Add some Greek yogurt or mayonnaise for extra creaminess. Pour the mixture into a salad bowl and top with avocado or cucumber slices. Mix roasted red peppers with Greek yogurt, garlic, and herbs such as parsley and basil. Served with whole wheat flatbread, carrot sticks and cucumber slices.

Berry Smoothie Bowl

Smoothie Bowls are a fun way to enjoy visually appealing and healthy snacks. Mix frozen berries with Greek yogurt, spinach and almond milk. Pour into a bowl and garnish with sliced bananas, chia seeds and granola. You can also add a little honey.

Roasted Chickpeas

Chickpeas are high in protein and fiber, making them a great healthy snack. Add olive oil and your favorite spices such as paprika, cumin and garlic powder. Bake in the oven and enjoy as a crunchy snack.

Caprese Skewer

Caprese Skewer is a simple, elegant appetizer that is also nutritious. Skewer alternating cherry tomatoes, fresh basil leaves, and small balls of fresh mozzarella. A drizzle of balsamic vinegar and olive oil adds flavor.

Whole Wheat Crisp Guacamole

Guacamole is a delicious, nutritious dip. Avocados are packed with healthy fats and antioxidants, while coriander and lime juice add flavor and freshness. Pair with whole wheat tortilla chips for a satisfying crunch.

Zucchini Fritters

Zucchini Fritters are a delicious and healthy way to sneak in some veggies. Mix large zucchini with whole grains, eggs, and herbs such as parsley and dill. Form into patties and fry in a little olive oil until golden brown. Serve with Greek yogurt or tzatziki sauce.

Seaweed Salad
Seaweed is a nutrient-rich food rich in minerals and antioxidants. Try making a simple nori salad with seaweed, sesame oil, rice vinegar, and sesame seeds. A unique and healthy appetizer that will impress your guests.

Watermelon Salad

Watermelon is a refreshing fruit rich in lycopene, a powerful antioxidant. Toss diced watermelon with feta cheese, mint leaves and a drizzle of balsamic vinegar—a sweet and savory salad perfect for summer.

Cucumber Cream Cheese Bites

Cucumber Cream Cheese Bites are a light, refreshing appetizer that's easy to make. Cut the cucumber into strips and sprinkle with plenty of cream cheese. A sprinkle of dill or chives adds flavor.

Roasted Beet and Goat Cheese Crostini

Beets are rich in antioxidants and add color to any dish. Roast the beets in the oven until tender and slice thinly. Spread goat cheese on slices of whole-wheat baguette and top with slices of beetroot. A touch of honey or balsamic glaze adds sweetness.

Roasted Eggplant Potato Chips

Eggplant is a versatile vegetable rich in fiber and antioxidants. Slice the eggplant thinly and toss with a little olive oil and your favorite spices such as garlic and paprika. Bake in the oven until crisp and enjoy as a healthy snack.

Chocolate Avocado Pudding

Chocolate Avocado Pudding is a rich, creamy and healthy dessert. Mix the avocado with cocoa powder, almond milk, and a sweetener such as honey or maple syrup. A delicious way to satisfy your sweet tooth while still getting healthy fats and antioxidants.
In summary, these cancer-fighting snacks and appetizers are not only delicious, they're packed with nutrients and antioxidants. Incorporating these foods into your diet can help support your body's defenses against cancer and improve your overall health and well-being.Enjoy these delicious treats while taking care of your body.

Chapter 7: Cancer-Fighting Smoothies and Juices

Smoothies and juices are a popular and convenient way to consume a wide variety of fruits, vegetables, and other cancer-fighting ingredients. They are also easy to digest and absorb, making them a great option for those undergoing cancer treatment who may have difficulty eating solid foods.

When making cancer-fighting smoothies and juices, it's important to choose ingredients that are high in antioxidants, anti-inflammatory compounds, and other nutrients that have been shown to have anti-cancer properties. Here are some of the best ingredients to include in your cancer-fighting smoothies and juices:

Leafy Greens: Leafy greens like kale, spinach, and Swiss chard are packed with cancer-fighting compounds like vitamin C, vitamin K, and beta-carotene. They also contain chlorophyll, which has been shown to help detoxify the body and reduce inflammation.

Berries: Berries like blueberries, strawberries, and raspberries are rich in antioxidants like anthocyanins, which have been shown to have anti-cancer properties. They are also low in sugar and high in fiber, making them a great choice for those watching their blood sugar levels.

Cruciferous Vegetables: Cruciferous vegetables like broccoli, cauliflower, and Brussels sprouts contain compounds called glucosinolate, which have been shown to have anti-cancer properties. They are also high in fiber and other nutrients that are important for overall health.

Turmeric: Turmeric contains a compound called curcumin, which has been shown to have potent anti-inflammatory and anti-cancer properties. It's important to note that curcumin is not well-absorbed by the body on its own, so it's best to consume turmeric with a source of fat and black pepper, which can help enhance its absorption.
Ginger: Ginger contains compounds called gingerol and shoals, which have been shown to have anti-inflammatory and anti-cancer properties. It's also great for digestion and can help soothe nausea, which is a common side effect of cancer treatment.

Now that you know some of the best cancer-fighting ingredients to include in your smoothies and juices, here are some recipes to get you started:

Recipe 1: Berry Blast Smoothie

Ingredients:

1 cup frozen mixed berries

1 banana

1 cup spinach

1/2 cup almond milk

1 tbsp chia seeds

1 tsp honey

Directions:

Add all ingredients to a blender and blend until smooth.

Pour into a glass and enjoy!

Recipe 2: Green Goddess Juice

Ingredients:

2 cups kale

1 cucumber

2 celery stalks

1 lemon
1-inch piece of ginger

1 green apple

Directions:

Wash and chop all ingredients.

Place ingredients from leafy greens to apple into juicer.

Pour into a glass and enjoy!

Recipe 3: Turmeric and Ginger Smoothie

Ingredients:

1 banana

1 cup almond milk
1 tsp turmeric

1/2 tsp ginger

1 tsp honey

1/4 tsp black pepper

Directions:

Place all ingredients in blender and blend until smooth.

Pour into a glass and enjoy!

When making cancer-fighting smoothies and juices, it's important to listen to your body and make adjustments as needed. If an ingredient doesn't work for you, try replacing it with something else. And always consult your doctor before changing your diet.

Anti-Cancer Smoothies and Juices can also support the body's natural detoxification processes. Many cancer treatments, such as chemotherapy and radiation, can damage healthy cells and tissues in the body. This damage can lead to the formation of free radicals, unstable molecules that can cause further damage and inflammation in the body.

Antioxidants, found in many ingredients in cancer-fighting smoothies and juices, can help neutralize these free radicals and reduce the damage they can cause. This can help support the body's natural detoxification processes and reduce inflammation, which can improve overall health and well-being.

In addition to choosing the right ingredients, there are a few other things to consider when making anti-cancer smoothies and juices. Here are some tips to help you get the most out of your cancer-fighting beverages:

Choose Organic Whenever Possible: When making smoothies and juices, it's important to choose organic ingredients. This can help reduce exposure to pesticides and other harmful chemicals that can contribute to cancer risk.

Use different colors: the lighter your smoothie or juice, the more nutrients it contains. Try adding different colors to your drinks to ensure you're getting a wide range of nutrients.
Watch out for sugar: While many fruits are naturally sweet, it's important to watch out for added sugar when preparing smoothies and juices. Too much sugar can contribute to inflammation and other health issues, so try to keep your added sugar intake to a minimum.

Experiment with Different Ingredients: Don't be afraid to experiment with different ingredients when making cancer-fighting smoothies and juices. There are so many fruits, vegetables, and other ingredients that can be used to make delicious and nutritious drinks.

Drink in moderation: While smoothies and juices are a great way to get extra nutrients, it's important to drink them in moderation. Consuming too many smoothies or juices can lead to excessive sugar intake and other health issues, so make sure to listen to your body and drink in moderation.

Finally, cancer-fighting smoothies and juices can be great additions to a healthy diet for those undergoing cancer treatment or looking to reduce their risk of cancer. By choosing the right ingredients and following a few simple tips, you can create delicious and nutritious beverages that support your overall health and well-being.

Chapter 8: Cancer-Fighting Desserts and Snacks

When it comes to desserts and snacks, many people feel that if they follow a cancer-fighting diet, they have to stop altogether. But it's not entirely true. While it's true that many desserts and treats contain sugar and unhealthy ingredients, which can increase inflammation and contribute to the growth of cancer, it's important to satisfy your sweet tooth without compromising your health.

In this chapter, we'll show you some cancer-fighting desserts and treats you can enjoy without feeling guilty.

Fruit Salad

Fruit Salad is perfect for those with a sweet tooth but want to avoid added sugar. Fruits contain antioxidants, fiber and vitamins that can help fight cancer and improve overall health.Combine your favorite fruits such as berries, apples, mangoes, kiwis and oranges, you can add chopped nuts and seeds for an even crunchier fruit salad.

Dark Chocolate

Dark chocolate is rich in flavonoids. Flavonoids are powerful antioxidants that help prevent cancer and reduce inflammation. Aim for dark chocolate with at least 70% cocoa and consume in moderation to avoid excess sugar and calories.

Chia Seeds

Chia Seeds are an excellent source of fiber, protein and healthy omega-3 fats, making them ideal ingredients for healthy desserts and snacks. Chia pudding is effortless to make by mixing chia seeds with your favorite milk, such as almond, coconut, or soy milk, and allowing it to sit for a few hours or overnight. You can add some fresh fruit or nuts to the top for added flavor and nutrition.

Baked Apples

Baked apples are a classic dessert that is easy to prepare and delicious to eat. Apples are rich in antioxidants and fiber, making them an excellent addition to a cancer-fighting diet. To make baked apples, cut the core out of an apple and stuff it with a mixture of oats, cinnamon, and chopped nuts. Bake in the oven until tender and serve warm with yogurt or whipped cream.

Sorbet

Sorbet is a refreshing and healthy alternative to sugary and unhealthy fatty ice cream. They make sorbets from fruit, sugar, and water, and are dairy-free and free of artificial ingredients.Mix your favorite fruits such as strawberries, mangoes, and peaches with a little water and sugar and freeze until firm to make sorbets.
Banana Ice Cream

Banana Ice Cream is a healthy alternative to regular ice cream that is easy to make at home. Puree frozen bananas with a little milk or yogurt until smooth and creamy and enjoy.You can add cocoa powder, vanilla extract, or nuts for added flavor and nutrition.

Bars

Granola bars are a great on-the-go snack that's easy to make at home. Homemade granola bars are healthier than store-bought versions that are high in sugar and unhealthy fats.You can combine oatmeal, nuts, seeds, and dried fruit and add honey or maple syrup to make granola bars. increase. Bake in the oven until golden brown and store in an airtight container for a quick and healthy snack.

A cancer-fighting diet doesn't mean you have to give up desserts and snacks altogether. Choosing healthy, nutritious foods can satisfy your sweet tooth while supporting your overall health and well-being. Try out these cancer-fighting desserts and treats and experiment with new recipes to find what works best for you. may seem counterintuitive, but there are actually many ways to enjoy these treats without compromising your health. By choosing ingredients rich in antioxidants, fiber, and other essential nutrients, you can enjoy desserts that actually help fight cancer and promote good health. One of the best ways to enjoy it is to make it at home. When preparing desserts, you have complete control over the ingredients and can choose to use whole, natural ingredients that are good for you.

Another great way to enjoy healthy desserts is to incorporate fresh fruits and vegetables. They packed fruits and vegetables with essential vitamins, minerals, and antioxidants, which can help reduce inflammation, fight cancer, and improve overall health. Berries, for example, are high in antioxidants, and can be added to smoothies, yogurt, or even eaten on their own as a healthy snack.

With sweeteners, it's best to avoid processed sugars, which can contribute to inflammation and increase the risk of cancer. Instead, try using natural sweeteners like honey, maple syrup, or stevia. These sweeteners are lower on the glycemic index and are less likely to cause a spike in blood sugar levels, which can be harmful to your health.

In addition to sweet treats, there are plenty of healthy snack options to satisfy your appetite without sacrificing your health. Some examples include roasted chickpeas, air popcorn, and sliced vegetables with hummus.
Ultimately, the key to enjoying healthy desserts and treats is to approach them in moderation. While it's important to indulge in the foods you love, it's also important to be mindful of how much and how often you consume them. By incorporating healthy desserts and treats into your diet in a balanced

way, you can support your health and wellness
while enjoying the foods you love.

Chapter 9: Cooking Tips for a Cancer-Fighting Diet

Cooking is an integral part of a cancer-fighting diet. It is the process by which food is prepared, cooked and served. However, not all cooking methods are created equal to retain the nutrients in food.

Use Healthy Fats

Cooking with Healthy Fats Essential in a cancer-fighting diet. Olive oil, avocado oil, and coconut oil are some examples of healthy fats that can be used in cooking. These oils have a high smoke point, which means they can withstand high temperatures without breaking down into harmful compounds. Avoid using vegetable oils or canola oil as they contain trans fats that can be harmful to your health.

Don't Overcook Vegetables

Overcooking vegetables can cause them to lose their cancer-fighting properties. I recommend you steam or stir-fry your vegetables to preserve their nutrients. You can also roast them in the oven with a bit of oil and seasoning. Boiling vegetables is not recommended as it can cause the nutrients to leach out into the water.

Choose Lean Proteins

For protein, choose lean options such as fish, chicken, and turkey. Red meat should be consumed in moderation, as it contains high levels of saturated fat. Processed meats such as bacon, sausages, and deli meats should be avoided altogether. When cooking meat, it is best to grill, broil, or bake rather than fry. I have. Garlic, turmeric, ginger, and cinnamon are examples of spices that have been shown to have anticancer properties.Fresh herbs such as parsley, basil, and thyme also have anticancer properties and add flavor to dishes. can do.

Eat a Variety of Fruits and Vegetables

Eating a variety of fruits and vegetables is important for getting a variety of nutrients that help fight cancer. Different colored fruits and vegetables contain different nutrients that help prevent cancer. For example, orange fruits and vegetables contain beta-carotene, which has been shown to reduce the risk of lung cancer. Grain grains are an excellent source of dietary fiber and nutrients. It also helps reduce the risk of cancer. Avoid refined grains such as white bread, white rice, and white pasta, as they strip nutrients during the refining process.

Avoid Processed Foods

Processed foods are high in salt, sugar and unhealthy fats. They are also low in nutrients and may contribute to the development of cancer. It's best to avoid processed foods entirely and opt for whole foods instead.

Use non-toxic cookware

The type of cookware you use can also affect your health. Nonstick cookware contains a chemical called perfluorooctanoic acid (PFOA) that has been linked to cancer. We recommend using stainless steel, cast iron, or ceramic cookware instead.

Practicing safe cooking

Practicing safe cooking also helps reduce the risk of cancer. Do not cook food at high temperatures or for long periods of time as it may form harmful compounds. Always use clean utensils and cutting boards to avoid cross-contamination.

Cooking is an integral part of a cancer-fighting diet. Use healthy fats, avoid overcooking vegetables, choose lean proteins such as spices and herbs, eat a variety of fruits and vegetables, choose whole grains, avoid processed foods, and use non-toxic cookware. You can stay healthy by using it and adopting safe cooking practices. To stay aware of the anti-cancer properties of the foods you eat.

In addition to these cooking tips, there are other things you can do to support your cancer-fighting diet. For example, incorporating regular exercise into your daily routine can reduce your risk of cancer and improve your overall health. It's also important to stay hydrated by drinking plenty of water throughout the day.

When it comes to meal planning, prepping meals ahead of time ensures that you have healthy options available throughout the week. You can also experiment with new recipes and flavors to make meals interesting and fun.
Finally, it's important to remember that no single food or nutrient will prevent or cure cancer. A cancer-fighting diet should be part of an overall

healthy lifestyle, including regular exercise, managing stress, and avoiding harmful behaviors such as smoking and excessive drinking.

In summary, a cancer-fighting diet can help reduce cancer risk and improve overall health. Incorporating these cooking tips into your daily routine can help preserve the cancer-fighting properties of the foods you eat and support your overall health and well-being.

Chapter 10: Maintaining a Cancer-Fighting Diet for Long-Term Health

Above all, it's important to understand that a cancer-fighting diet is not a one-time fix. It is a lifestyle change that must be followed in the long term. Even if you get great results in a short period of time, returning to old habits will only bring back old problems. Therefore, it is important to make this meal part of your daily routine.

Keep a food diary

One of the best ways to keep a cancer-fighting diet is to keep a food diary. This will help you keep track of what and how much you ate. You can also watch your calorie intake and avoid overeating. This way you can make sure you are sticking to your diet and make changes accordingly. can throw you off balance. It is important to have a regular meal plan and stick to it. Fewer and more meals a day are more effective than large meals. This slows down your metabolism and provides a steady flow of energy to your body.

Avoid Processed Foods

Processed foods contain preservatives, additives and chemicals that are harmful to your health in the long term. Instead, choose fresh, whole foods that are packed with nutrients and antioxidants. Fruits, vegetables, whole grains and lean proteins should be the mainstays of your diet.

Hydration

Water is essential for our bodies to function properly. Drinking plenty of water throughout the day is important to keep your body hydrated. Avoid sugary and carbonated drinks as they add unnecessary calories and can be detrimental to your health.

1 Watch Your Serving Sizes

1 Serving Sizes Play An Important Role In Maintaining A Healthy Weight. Even if you eat healthy food, you will get excess calories if you eat too much. It's important to be mindful of portion sizes and not overeat.

Treat yourself moderately

It's okay to eat your favorite treat once in a while. However, it is important to do this in moderation. A small portion of ice cream or cake once in a while is not harmful to your health. However, regular consumption of these treats adds unnecessary calories and can be detrimental to your health. There are no elements. It's important to stay active and exercise regularly. You don't have to go to the gym every day, but you can keep fit by incorporating physical activity into your daily routine.

Don't Blame Yourself

Finally, it's important to be kind to yourself. Don't blame yourself for eating unhealthy foods or skipping workouts by mistake. Instead, forgive yourself and get back on track. Remember that staying on a cancer-fighting diet is a journey, and there will be challenges along the way. It is a lifestyle initiative. By choosing a healthy diet, staying active, and paying attention to your habits, you can maintain your diet and reap benefits for years to come. Remember that leading a healthy lifestyle isn't just about looking better, it's about feeling better, having more energy, and reducing your risk of chronic diseases like cancer. By following the tips in this chapter, you can make cancer-fighting meals part of your daily routine and reap the long-term health benefits.

It's important to remember that lifestyle changes aren't always easy and it's okay to struggle. However, it's important to stay motivated and focus on the long-term benefits of a healthy lifestyle. Surround yourself with a support system that encourages you to make healthy choices and stay on course.

In addition to the tips above, it's important to stay up to date with the latest research in cancer prevention and treatment. As new information becomes available, it is important to adjust your diet and lifestyle to reflect the latest research.Read reputable sources and consult your doctor to stay informed. please.

It's important to remember that a cancer-fighting diet is only part of a healthy lifestyle. Other factors such as stress management, sleep and social support also play an important role in maintaining good health. Taking a holistic approach to health and well-being can maximize your chances of living a long and healthy life.

In summary, a cancer-fighting diet for long-term health requires a commitment to making healthy food choices, staying active, and watching your habits. By making these changes a part of your daily routine and staying motivated, you'll reap the long-term benefits of a healthy lifestyle. Remember, a healthy lifestyle is a journey, not a destination.

Conclusion

In summary, a cancer-fighting diet is more than just a diet, it's a lifestyle change. It's a commitment to making healthy choices that can have a big impact on your health and well-being. It can improve your overall health and improve your quality of life.

This book explores the science behind cancer-fighting diets, foods and nutrients that may help prevent cancer, and practical steps to incorporate these foods into your diet. . We also discussed the importance of exercise, stress management and social support in maintaining a healthy lifestyle.

But this book is more than just a collection of tips and advice. It's a call to action. A reminder that we have the power to control our health and well-being. We don't have to be passive cancer victims. We can take steps to prevent this and fight back once they diagnose us.

Cancer-fighting diets are not silver bullets. It's not a panacea for cancer. But it is a powerful tool that can change our lives. Making healthy choices can increase your chances of avoiding cancer and living a longer, healthier life. You can also set an example for your friends and family by making these choices. You can show that a healthy lifestyle is not only possible, but fun. We can inspire them to change their lives and help create a healthier and happier world. increase. Use the knowledge and insights you gain here and put them into practice. Changing your diet and lifestyle can have a big impact on your health. And share your knowledge with others. Spread the word about cancer-fighting diets and encourage others to take care of their health.

Remember, the power to prevent cancer is in our hands. Let's use it to create a healthier and better future for ourselves and the next generation.